Depression in Kids

A Comprehensive Guide to Understanding and Treating Childhood Depression

STEPHEN K. DAY

Copyright ©2023, Stephen K. Day

All rights reserved.

No part of this book may be reproduced or transmitted in any form or by any means, electronic or mechanical, including photocopying, recording, or by any information storage and retrieval system, without permission in writing from the publisher.

TABLE OF CONTENTS

INTRODUCTION

Childhood depression is a serious and often misunderstood mental health condition that affects children of all ages and can have a significant impact on their development, relationships, and overall well-being.

It is characterized by persistent feelings of sadness, irritability, loss of interest in activities and hobbies that the child previously enjoyed, changes in appetite and sleep patterns, difficulty concentrating, low energy and fatigue, and sometimes even thoughts of death or suicide.

These symptoms can interfere with a child's ability to function in school, at home, and in social situations and can lead to problems with grades, relationships with peers and family members, and overall quality of life.

Childhood depression can range in severity from mild to severe and may be triggered by a variety of factors, including genetics, brain chemistry, family dynamics, life events and stressors, and other health conditions.

It is important to recognize the signs of childhood depression and seek treatment as soon as possible, as untreated depression can lead to long-term complications and may interfere with a child's development and ability to reach their full potential.

Treatment for childhood depression typically involves a combination of therapies, such as cognitive-behavioral therapy, family therapy, and medication, as well as support and guidance from mental health professionals and caregivers. With the right support and treatment, children with depression can learn to manage their symptoms and lead healthy, happy lives.

It is important to note that childhood depression is not simply a normal part of growing up or a phase that children will eventually outgrow. It is a serious and potentially life-threatening condition that requires professional treatment.

If you suspect that your child may be experiencing depression, it is important to speak with a mental health professional or your child's healthcare provider as soon as possible to discuss treatment options and get the support and care your child needs.

Prevalence Of Childhood Depression

Childhood depression is a serious and potentially debilitating mental health disorder that affects a significant number of children and adolescents. According to the National Institute of Mental Health (NIMH), an estimated 2-3% of children in the United States experience depression at some point during their childhood, although the actual prevalence may be higher due to underdiagnosis.

Depression is more common in girls than in boys, with a female-to-male ratio of approximately 2:1. It can occur at any age, although it is most commonly diagnosed in adolescents.

Children with depression may experience a wide range of symptoms, including persistent sadness or irritability, loss of interest in activities they previously enjoyed, changes in appetite or sleep patterns, difficulty concentrating, low energy or fatigue, and thoughts of death or suicide.

These symptoms can have significant impacts on a child's overall well-being and development, and they may interfere with their ability to function at home, school, and in social settings.

It is important for parents and caregivers to be aware of the signs and symptoms of childhood depression and to seek help from a mental health professional if they are concerned about their child's mental health. Early identification and treatment of depression in children is essential for improving outcomes and helping children recover and go on to lead healthy and fulfilling lives. There are a variety of treatment options available for children with depression, including therapy, medication, and a combination of both. With proper treatment, children with depression can learn coping skills and develop healthy ways of managing their emotions, thoughts, and behaviors, and they can experience significant improvement in their symptoms and overall functioning.

There are several risk factors that may increase a child's risk for developing depression. These include having a family history of depression, being exposed to stress or trauma, having low self-esteem, being a perfectionist, and having certain medical conditions. Children who have experienced significant life changes, such as a loss or a move, may also be at increased risk for depression.

Having a family history of depression means that a child may be more likely to experience it themselves due to genetic factors or environmental influences in the family.

Exposure to stress or trauma, such as abuse, neglect, or a natural disaster, can disrupt a child's sense of safety and security and lead to ongoing feelings of anxiety and sadness. Children with low self-esteem may have negative thoughts about themselves and their abilities, which can become self-fulfilling and lead to a downward spiral of negative emotions and behaviors. Perfectionism can lead to feelings of inadequacy and disappointment when a child is unable to meet their own high standards or the expectations of others, and may contribute to a negative self-image. Certain medical conditions, such as chronic pain or a learning disability, can impact a child's daily life and lead to feelings of frustration or helplessness.

It is important to identify and address these risk factors in order to prevent or mitigate the development of depression in children. This may involve seeking professional help, such as therapy or medication, as well as providing support and understanding to the child as they navigate these challenges.

CHAPTER 1: SYMPTOMS OF CHILDHOOD DEPRESSION

Physical Symptoms

Children with depression may experience a range of physical symptoms that can significantly impact their overall health and well-being. These physical symptoms may include changes in appetite and weight, either an increase or decrease, as well as sleep disturbances such as difficulty falling asleep or staying asleep, or excessive sleepiness during the day.

Children with depression may also feel fatigued and have low energy levels, which can make it difficult for them to engage in activities that they normally enjoy, such as participating in sports or spending time with friends. In addition to these symptoms, children with depression may also experience physical aches and pains, such as headaches or stomachaches, that have no apparent cause.

These physical symptoms may be a result of the changes in brain chemistry and hormone levels that occur with depression, as the disorder can affect the body's systems and functions in a number of ways.

Alternatively, these physical symptoms may be a response to the emotional and behavioral changes that often accompany depression, such as feelings of sadness, hopelessness, and low self-esteem, as well as changes in social and cognitive functioning. Children with depression may also experience changes in their energy level, motivation, and concentration, which can further contribute to the development of physical symptoms.

Regardless of the cause, it is important to address these physical symptoms as part of a comprehensive treatment plan for children with depression, in order to improve their overall health and quality of life.

This may involve a combination of medications, such as antidepressants, and therapy, such as cognitive-behavioral therapy or interpersonal therapy, to address the underlying causes of the disorder and help children learn coping skills to manage their symptoms. It is also important for parents and caregivers to be supportive and provide a safe and nurturing environment for children with depression to help them feel loved and valued.

Emotional Symptoms

Emotional symptoms of childhood depression can be persistent and can significantly impact a child's daily life. These symptoms can include persistent sadness or irritability, feelings of hopelessness or worthlessness, difficulty concentrating, a loss of interest in activities that were previously enjoyable, and difficulty experiencing pleasure or happiness.

Persistent sadness or irritability may manifest as a child feeling down or unhappy most of the time, or they may experience mood swings and feel easily annoyed or frustrated. These emotions can be intense and difficult to shake, and they can interfere with a child's ability to enjoy activities or interact with others.

Feelings of hopelessness or worthlessness may lead a child to believe that things will never get better or that they are not good enough or worthy of love and attention. These negative beliefs can be pervasive and can lead to a child feeling helpless or defeated.

Difficulty concentrating can impact a child's performance in school or other activities and can lead to feelings of frustration or overwhelm. A child may struggle to focus on tasks or to remember things, which can interfere with their daily functioning.

A loss of interest in activities that were previously enjoyable can be a significant

change for a child and can lead to feelings of isolation or loneliness. A child may lose interest in hobbies, sports, or social activities that they used to enjoy, which can be a source of sadness.

Difficulty experiencing pleasure or happiness may manifest as a lack of emotional expression or a sense that a child is just going through the motions of life rather than truly living it. This can be a source of frustration and sadness for a child.

It is important to note that every child is different and may experience different symptoms of depression. It is also possible for a child to experience some of these symptoms without having depression. If you are concerned about your child's emotional well-being, it is important to seek the advice of a mental health professional.

Behavioral Symptoms

Children with depression may exhibit a wide range of behavioral changes that can impact their daily lives and relationships. These changes can include isolating themselves from family and friends, withdrawing from social activities and hobbies that they previously enjoyed, and experiencing significant changes in their school performance.

In addition to these behaviors, children with depression may also engage in risky or reckless behaviors, such as reckless driving or engaging in dangerous activities. These behaviors can be a way for children to cope with the negative emotions and feelings that they are experiencing as a result of their depression.

It is important to recognize and address these behavioral changes in children, as they can have serious consequences for their physical and emotional health and well-being. If left unchecked, these behaviors can lead to further problems, such as substance abuse, self-harm, and other mental health issues. It is essential to seek help from a mental health professional if you are concerned about your child's behavior.

A mental health professional can help to identify the underlying cause of the behavior and provide the necessary support and treatment to help your child overcome their depression and regain their mental health and well-being. It is important to remember that with the right treatment and support, children with depression can recover and go on to lead healthy, fulfilling lives.

CHAPTER 2: CAUSES OF CHILDHOOD DEPRESSION

Biological Factors

There are several biological factors that may contribute to the development of childhood depression. These include genetics, hormonal imbalances, and changes in brain chemistry. Understanding these factors can help us better understand the causes of depression and how it may be treated.

Genetics

Children who have a family history of depression may be at increased risk for developing the condition themselves, as there may be a genetic component to the disorder. This means that individuals may be more likely to develop depression if they have a parent or other close relative who has experienced the disorder. Studies have shown that genetics can play a role in the development of depression, although the exact extent of this influence is not yet fully understood.

It is thought that multiple genes may be involved in the development of depression, and that these genes may interact with environmental factors to increase the risk of the disorder.

Some studies have found that certain genetic variations may be associated with an increased risk of depression, while others have found no such association. It is likely that genetics plays a complex role in the development of the disorder, and more research is needed to fully understand this relationship.

Hormonal imbalances

Hormonal imbalances, such as those that occur during puberty, may also contribute to the development of depression. The hormonal changes that occur during puberty can sometimes lead to mood changes and emotional instability, which may increase the risk of developing depression.

For example, low levels of estrogen, a hormone that plays a role in regulating mood and emotion, have been linked to an increased risk of depression. Other hormones that may be involved in the development of depression include thyroid hormones, which play a role in regulating metabolism and energy levels, and cortisol, a hormone that is produced in response to stress.

Changes in brain chemistry

Changes in brain chemistry, including the levels of certain neurotransmitters, may also play a role in the development of depression. Neurotransmitters are chemicals that help transmit messages between brain cells, and imbalances in their levels can affect mood and emotional regulation. For example, low levels of serotonin, a neurotransmitter that plays a role in regulating mood, have been linked to depression.

Other neurotransmitters that may be involved in the development of depression include dopamine and norepinephrine. Some studies have found that individuals with depression have abnormal levels of these neurotransmitters in their brains, while others have found no such abnormalities. It is likely that the relationship between neurotransmitter levels and depression is complex and not fully understood.

It is important to note that these are just a few of the many potential biological factors that may contribute to the development of childhood depression. Other potential factors may include medical conditions, physical or sexual abuse, and other life stressors. The development of depression is often the result of a combination of these and other factors, and each person's experience with the disorder may be unique.

Environmental Factors

Environmental factors that may contribute to the development of childhood depression include exposure to stress or trauma, lack of social support, and significant life changes. Children who have experienced abuse, neglect, or other forms of trauma may be at increased risk for developing depression, as this type of experience can cause long-term changes in brain development and function.

These changes can affect the way the brain regulates emotions and responds to stress, making it more difficult for children to cope with challenges and setbacks. In addition, children who lack supportive relationships or a sense of belonging may be more vulnerable to developing depression, as these types of social connections can provide a sense of security and help to buffer against stress.

Children who do not have access to supportive relationships may feel isolated and alone, which can increase the risk of depression. Similarly, children who do not have a sense of belonging or connection to a larger community may feel disconnected and unsupported, which can also increase the risk of depression.

Finally, children who have experienced significant life changes, such as the loss of a loved one or a move to a new home, may also be at increased risk for developing depression, as these types of events can be emotionally taxing and disrupt established routines and support systems.

It is important to note that these are just some of the many potential environmental risk factors for childhood depression, and that the development of depression is likely influenced by a complex interaction of multiple factors.

Psychological Factors

Childhood depression is a serious and complex mental health condition that can have a significant impact on a child's overall well-being and development. It is characterized by persistent feelings of sadness, hopelessness, and a lack of interest or pleasure in activities that were previously enjoyable.

While the exact causes of childhood depression are not fully understood, research suggests that a combination of genetic, environmental, and psychological factors may contribute to its development.

One key psychological factor that may increase

the risk of childhood depression is negative thought patterns. These refer to the way an individual thinks about themselves, others, and the world around them. Children who engage in negative self-talk, such as thinking that they are not good enough or that they will never be successful, may be more vulnerable to developing depression.

Negative thought patterns can also include negative beliefs about oneself, such as believing that one is unlovable or unworthy, or negative beliefs about the world, such as believing that life is always unfair or that nothing will ever go well. These negative thoughts can become ingrained over time and can be difficult to change, making them a significant risk factor for depression.

Low self-esteem is another psychological factor that may contribute to the development of childhood depression. Children with low self-esteem may feel inadequate or unworthy, and may struggle to feel good about themselves or their accomplishments. They may also have difficulty standing up for themselves or believing in their own abilities, which can lead to feelings of helplessness and hopelessness. Children with low self-esteem may also be more prone to bullying or social isolation, which can further increase the risk of depression.

Perfectionism, or the belief that one must be perfect in order to be accepted or valued, may also contribute to the development of depression in children.

Children who are perfectionistic may feel constant pressure to meet unrealistic standards, which can lead to feelings of inadequacy and failure. They may also struggle to enjoy activities or hobbies because they are too focused on achieving perfection, which can further contribute to feelings of unhappiness and dissatisfaction. Perfectionistic children may also have difficulty seeking help or support when they are struggling, as they may believe that they should be able to handle everything on their own.

In addition to these psychological factors, other risk factors for childhood depression may include a family history of depression, exposure to traumatic events or chronic stress, and certain medical conditions or medications.

It is important for parents, caregivers, and other loved ones to be aware of these risk factors and to seek appropriate help if they suspect that a child may be struggling with depression.

Early intervention can be critical in helping children overcome depression and go on to lead healthy, fulfilling lives. This may involve a combination of therapy, medication, and other supportive interventions, depending on the specific needs of the child.

CHAPTER 3: DIAGNOSIS OF CHILDHOOD DEPRESSION

Assessing For Depression in Children

The process of diagnosing childhood depression involves a comprehensive evaluation of the child's physical, emotional, and behavioral symptoms. A healthcare provider will typically begin by conducting a thorough physical examination and medical history in order to rule out any underlying medical conditions that may be causing the child's symptoms.

This may include asking about the child's symptoms, as well as their family history, medical history, and any other relevant information. The provider may also ask the child about their daily routine, including their sleep patterns, appetite, energy levels, and activities.

During the physical examination, the healthcare provider will carefully assess the child's overall physical health and check for any signs of illness or injury that may be affecting their mental health. They may also ask the child about any physical symptoms they are experiencing, such as fatigue, headaches, or stomachaches, which could be related to depression.

In addition to the physical examination and medical history, the healthcare provider may also ask the child to complete a depression screening tool or questionnaire. These tools are designed to help identify symptoms of depression and assess the severity of the condition. Some common screening tools for childhood depression include the Children's Depression Inventory (CDI) and the Mood and Feelings Questionnaire (MFQ). The healthcare provider may also ask the child to complete other psychological assessments or cognitive tests to further assess their mental health.

The healthcare provider may also ask the child's parents or caregivers about their observations of the child's behavior and functioning. It is important for the provider to gather as much information as possible in order to accurately diagnose and treat the child's condition.

If the healthcare provider determines that the child is experiencing depression, they may recommend a combination of treatments, such as therapy, medication, and lifestyle changes, to help the child manage their symptoms and improve their overall mental health. These treatments may be provided by a team of healthcare professionals, including a child and adolescent psychiatrist, a psychologist, and a primary care physician. Working together, this team can help the child and their family develop a treatment plan that is tailored to their specific needs and goals.

Differential Diagnosis

Accurately identifying and distinguishing depression from other conditions that may present with similar symptoms is crucial for ensuring that individuals receive the most appropriate and effective treatment. Some conditions that may cause symptoms similar to depression include anxiety disorders, attention deficit hyperactivity disorder (ADHD), and certain medical conditions.

It is essential for healthcare providers to consider these possibilities during the assessment and evaluation process for a child who may be experiencing symptoms of depression. In order to make an accurate diagnosis, the healthcare provider may need to refer the child for additional testing or evaluation. This may include psychological evaluations, cognitive and developmental assessments, and physical examinations to rule out any underlying medical conditions.

The healthcare provider may also need to gather detailed information about the child's medical and mental health history, including any previous diagnoses and treatment received. They may also ask about the child's current symptoms, how long they have been present, and any factors that may be contributing to or exacerbating the symptoms.

It is also worth noting that comorbidity, or the presence of multiple mental health conditions simultaneously, is not uncommon. Therefore, it is important for healthcare providers to consider the possibility of coexisting conditions and to take a comprehensive approach to treatment.

This may involve coordinating care with multiple specialists and utilizing a range of treatment modalities, such as therapy, medication, and lifestyle modifications. By accurately diagnosing and treating all relevant conditions, the child can receive the most effective and comprehensive care possible.

Diagnostic Criteria for Childhood Depression

In order to be diagnosed with childhood depression, a child must meet the diagnostic criteria set forth in the Diagnostic and Statistical Manual of Mental Disorders (DSM-5).

These criteria include the presence of symptoms such as persistent sadness or irritability, loss of interest in activities that the child previously enjoyed, changes in appetite, sleep patterns, or energy levels, and difficulty concentrating or making decisions. These symptoms must be present for at least two weeks and must interfere with the child's ability to function in their daily life. The healthcare provider will consider the severity and duration of the symptoms in making a diagnosis of depression.

It is important to note that experiencing some of these symptoms occasionally is a normal part of life, but when they are persistent and interfere with daily functioning, it may be indicative of a more serious issue such as depression. Children with depression may also experience physical symptoms such as headaches, stomach aches, and fatigue, as well as behavioral changes such as increased irritability or aggression. They may also have difficulty functioning at school or in social situations, and may have a negative outlook on life.

It is also important to note that a diagnosis of depression should not be made lightly, and a thorough evaluation by a qualified healthcare professional is necessary to accurately diagnose and treat depression in children. This may include a physical examination, a review of the child's medical and family history, and psychological testing to rule out other potential causes of the child's symptoms.

In addition to a diagnosis, the healthcare provider may recommend treatment options such as therapy, medication, or a combination of both, depending on the severity of the child's symptoms and the individual needs of the child.

It is important to recognize that childhood depression is a serious condition that requires proper diagnosis and treatment. If you are concerned that your child may be experiencing depression, it is important to seek help from a qualified healthcare professional. With the right treatment, children with depression can improve their symptoms and lead fulfilling and healthy lives.

Medications

Antidepressant medications are a commonly used treatment for children and adolescents who are experiencing depression. These medications work by altering the balance of certain chemicals in the brain known as neurotransmitters, which are involved in mood regulation and other functions. There are several different classes of antidepressant medications, including selective serotonin reuptake inhibitors (SSRIs), tricyclic antidepressants, and monoamine oxidase inhibitors (MAOIs).

The healthcare provider will consider the child's specific symptoms, medical history, and other factors in selecting the most appropriate medication.

It is important to understand that antidepressant medications may take several weeks to become fully effective in reducing symptoms of depression. This is because the brain and its chemistry do not change overnight, and it takes time for the medication to reach therapeutic levels in the body and for the brain to adapt to the changes brought about by the medication. The child's healthcare provider may also adjust the dosage of the medication over time to find the most effective dose.

It is also important to closely monitor the child while they are taking antidepressants, as there is a risk of side effects and the possibility of worsening depression or suicidal thoughts. Common side effects of antidepressant medications may include nausea, headache, dizziness, dry mouth, and sleep problems. It is essential for the child to continue taking the medication as prescribed, even if they start to feel better, as abruptly stopping antidepressant medication can cause withdrawal symptoms and may lead to a relapse of depression.

In addition to taking medication, it is often recommended that children with depression also receive therapy or counseling to address the underlying causes of their depression and to learn coping skills.

This can be done through individual therapy, family therapy, or group therapy, and may involve techniques such as cognitive-behavioral therapy, dialectical behavior therapy, or interpersonal therapy. Therapy can help the child to learn healthy ways of managing their emotions and thoughts, and to develop positive coping strategies for dealing with stress and challenges.

It is important for parents and caregivers to

closely communicate with the child's healthcare provider about the potential risks and benefits of taking antidepressant medication, and to closely monitor the child's progress and any side effects.

It is also essential for the family to provide a supportive and nurturing environment for the child, as this can help to promote healing and recovery from depression. This may involve providing the child with a regular routine, encouraging them to engage in activities they enjoy, and offering emotional support and understanding.

Psychotherapy

Childhood depression is a serious mental health disorder that can significantly impact a child's quality of life and overall functioning. It is characterized by persistent feelings of sadness, low energy, difficulty concentrating, and changes in appetite, sleep patterns, and energy levels. Children with depression may also have difficulty with school, friendships, and other aspects of their daily lives.

Psychotherapy, also known as talk therapy, is a widely accepted and effective treatment for childhood depression. It involves working with a trained mental health professional to explore and address thoughts, feelings, and behaviors that may be causing difficulties in a child's life. There are several types of psychotherapy that can be helpful in treating childhood depression, including cognitive-behavioral therapy (CBT), interpersonal therapy, and family therapy.

Cognitive-behavioral therapy (CBT) is a type of psychotherapy that helps children identify and change negative thought patterns and behaviors that may be contributing to their depression. For example, a child who consistently thinks "I'm not good enough" or "I'm a failure" may feel discouraged and depressed. CBT can help the child learn to challenge these negative thoughts and recognize that they are not necessarily accurate or helpful. It can also teach children coping skills to help them better manage their emotions and behavior.

Interpersonal therapy is another form of psychotherapy that focuses on the child's relationships and communication skills. This approach may be particularly helpful in addressing issues that may be contributing to the child's depression, such as conflicts with peers or family members, social isolation, or poor communication skills. Interpersonal therapy can help the child learn how to express their feelings and needs more effectively, build stronger relationships, and improve their communication skills.

Family therapy is another treatment option that can be helpful in improving communication and problem-solving within the family system. When depression is impacting the child's relationships with family members, family therapy can be especially useful in helping the child and their family learn how to support one another and work through conflicts and challenges.

It is important to note that while psychotherapy can be an effective treatment for childhood depression, it is not always the best option for every child. Some children may benefit more from other treatments, such as medication or a combination of therapy and medication. It is important to work with a trained mental health professional to determine the best course of treatment for a child experiencing depression. The mental health professional will take into account the child's individual needs and circumstances, as well as the preferences of the child and their family, when developing a treatment plan.

Alternative And Complementary Treatments

In addition to traditional treatment methods like medication and psychotherapy, there are several alternative and complementary treatments that may be beneficial in the treatment of childhood depression. These treatments can be used in conjunction with traditional methods or as standalone treatments, depending on the individual needs and preferences of the child and their healthcare provider.

One such alternative treatment is exercise, which has been shown to be effective in reducing the symptoms of depression in adults and children alike. Regular physical activity can improve mood, reduce anxiety and stress, and increase feelings of self-worth and self-esteem. This can be especially important for children, as it can provide a sense of accomplishment and boost confidence.

Exercise can also have other physical and mental health benefits, such as improved sleep, increased energy levels, and stronger bones and muscles. There are many different types of exercise that can be beneficial for children, including sports, dancing, swimming, and running. It is important to find activities that the child enjoys and that are appropriate for their age and ability level. It can be helpful to set goals for exercise, such as increasing the duration or intensity of workouts over time, or trying new activities to keep things interesting.

Another alternative treatment is nutrition. A healthy, balanced diet can support overall physical and mental well-being, and may be particularly important for children with depression. Some research suggests that certain nutrients, such as omega-3 fatty acids and folate, may be particularly beneficial for mood. It is important to include a variety of fruits, vegetables, whole grains, lean proteins, and healthy fats in the child's diet to ensure that they are getting the nutrients they need.

It can be helpful to work with a healthcare provider or nutritionist to create a meal plan that is tailored to the child's specific needs. It may also be helpful to limit or eliminate processed foods, sugary drinks, and other unhealthy choices, as these can contribute to feelings of low mood and poor mental health.

Mindfulness practices, such as meditation or yoga, can also be useful in treating childhood depression. These practices can help children to develop skills like self-awareness, self-regulation, and stress management, which can be helpful in managing the symptoms of depression.

Mindfulness practices can also help children to better understand and manage their emotions, which can be especially important for those struggling with depression. These practices can be incorporated into daily routines, such as taking a few minutes to focus on the breath during bedtime or setting aside time for a guided meditation session. It is important to note that these practices should be introduced and supervised by a trained professional to ensure that they are used safely and effectively.

Overall, it is important to discuss all treatment options with a healthcare provider to determine the best course of action for the individual child. It is also important to remember that treatment for childhood depression may involve a combination of different approaches and may take time to be fully effective.

It is important to be patient and to work closely with the healthcare team to ensure that the child receives the support and care they need. It may also be helpful for the child to have support from friends and family, and to have a network of people they can turn to for help and encouragement.

CHAPTER 5: COPING WITH CHILDHOOD DEPRESSION

Strategies For Parents and Caregivers

Caring for a child with depression can be a challenging and often overwhelming experience for parents and caregivers. It requires a great deal of patience, understanding, and emotional strength to support a child who is struggling with this mental health condition.

It is important to remember that as a caregiver, it is crucial to prioritize your own self-care in order to be able to effectively support the child. This may include seeking support from family and friends, participating in activities that bring joy and relaxation, and seeking professional help if needed.

It is important to keep in mind that caring for a child with depression can be emotionally and physically draining. It is normal to feel overwhelmed and exhausted at times, and it is important to take breaks and practice self-care in order to maintain your own well-being.

This may involve seeking support from loved ones, taking time for yourself, and seeking professional help if needed. It is also important to remember that seeking support is not a sign of weakness, but rather a necessary step in taking care of oneself and being able to effectively support the child with depression.

In addition to seeking support and practicing self-care, it is important to educate oneself about depression and how to support a child who is struggling with it. This may involve learning about the different symptoms of depression, the different treatment options available, and how to communicate with the child about their feelings and experiences. It is also important to be patient and understanding with the child, as recovery from depression can be a long and difficult process.

It can be helpful to create a supportive and nurturing environment for the child, as this can help them feel safe and loved. This may involve spending quality time with the child, engaging in activities that they enjoy, and providing a sense of structure and stability in their daily routine. It is also important to be mindful of the child's physical and emotional needs, and to provide them with the resources and support they need to manage their depression.

Overall, caring for a child with depression requires a lot of patience, understanding, and emotional strength. It is important to prioritize self-care and seek support when needed in order to effectively support the child and help them manage their depression. With the right support and treatment, children with depression can learn to manage their symptoms and lead fulfilling lives.

Helping A Child with Depression

There are several strategies that parents and caregivers can use to help a child with depression. It is important to approach the child with empathy, understanding, and a willingness to listen and support them. Here are some specific tips for helping a child with depression:

Encourage open communication

Encourage the child to express their feelings and concerns openly and honestly. Let them know that it is okay to talk about their feelings and that you are there to listen. Make it a regular practice to check in with the child about how they are feeling and encourage them to share their thoughts and emotions. It can also be helpful to let the child know that they can come to you at any time to talk about their feelings.

Be an active listener

When the child talks to you, really listen to what they are saying. Avoid interrupting or trying to solve their problems right away. Just listen and show that you care. Reflect back on what the child has told you to show that you understand and are paying attention. Avoid minimizing their feelings or telling them to just "snap out of it." Instead, validate their emotions and let them know that it is normal to feel sad or overwhelmed at times.

Provide a supportive and understanding environment

Create a safe, supportive space for the child to talk about their feelings and concerns. Avoid judgment or criticism, and try to be understanding of their experiences. It can be helpful to validate their feelings and let them know that it is normal to feel sad or overwhelmed at times. Show support and encouragement by spending quality time with the child and participating in activities that they enjoy.

Encourage healthy habits

Help the child develop healthy habits such as regular exercise, a healthy diet, and getting enough sleep. These habits can help improve mood and overall well-being. Encourage the child to participate in activities that they enjoy, as this can help boost their mood and sense of accomplishment.

It can also be helpful to set limits on screen time and encourage the child to engage in activities that involve social interaction and human connection, such as joining a club or team.

Establish a routine

A regular routine can provide structure and consistency for the child, which can be helpful in managing depression. This may include setting a consistent bedtime, establishing a daily routine for meals and activities, and setting aside regular time for relaxation and self-care. It can be helpful to involve the child in creating their own routine and setting goals for themselves.

Be patient

Recovery from depression can be a slow process. It is important to be patient and to recognize that it may take time for the child to feel better. Encourage the child to take small steps towards improvement, and celebrate their progress along the way. It is also important to be patient with yourself as a parent or caregiver and to take care of your own mental health.

Seek professional help

If the child's symptoms persist or are severe, it may be helpful to enlist the support of a healthcare provider or mental health professional. They can help develop a treatment plan that is tailored to the child's specific needs.

This may include therapy, medication, or a combination of both. It is important to work with a professional who is experienced in treating children and adolescents with depression. Do not be afraid to seek help if you are worried about the child's mental health. The sooner you seek treatment, the better the chances of a successful outcome.

CHAPTER 6: PREVENTION OF CHILDHOOD DEPRESSION

Promoting Mental Health in Children

Mental health is an essential aspect of overall well-being and can have a significant impact on a child's development. It is important for parents and caregivers to prioritize the promotion of mental health in children and to be proactive in helping to prevent the development of conditions such as depression.

There are several ways in which parents and caregivers can support the mental health of their children. Building resilience, which is the ability to adapt and recover from difficult situations, is one important aspect. This can be achieved by teaching coping skills, such as deep breathing and mindfulness techniques, and fostering a positive outlook on life. Building resilience helps children to develop the skills and strategies they need to navigate challenges and setbacks, and to bounce back from adversity.

Creating a supportive and nurturing environment is also crucial for the mental health of children. This involves showing love, care, and attention, and setting clear boundaries and expectations. It is important to create a sense of safety and security, as children who feel secure are more likely to develop healthy mental habits. Providing a supportive environment can help children to feel valued and accepted, and to develop a sense of self-worth.

Teaching healthy communication and problem-solving skills can also be beneficial in promoting mental health. This includes teaching children how to express their emotions in a healthy way, how to listen actively, and how to work through conflicts in a constructive manner. Teaching these skills can help children to develop healthy relationships, to better understand and manage their emotions, and to resolve conflicts effectively.

Encouraging children to engage in activities that they enjoy, such as hobbies or sports, can also be helpful in promoting mental health. Participating in activities that bring joy and a sense of accomplishment can boost self-esteem and provide a sense of purpose. In addition, participating in social activities that promote a sense of belonging and connection, such as joining a club or team, can also be beneficial in this regard. Being part of a group can help children to feel supported and connected, and can foster a sense of community and belonging.

It is important to remember that every child is unique and may require different approaches to support their mental health. It is crucial for parents and caregivers to be attuned to the needs of their children and to seek out professional help if needed. This may include seeking guidance from a mental health professional, such as a child psychologist or counselor, who can provide specialized support and interventions.

By taking a proactive approach to promoting mental health, parents and caregivers can help their children to develop healthy habits and to thrive.

Identifying And Addressing Risk Factors

Depression is a serious mental health disorder that can have a significant impact on a child's overall well-being and development. Identifying and addressing risk factors for depression in children is crucial in order to prevent the development of this disorder and to support the mental health and well-being of children.

There are several steps that can be taken to reduce the risk of depression in children and to provide support and resources to those who may be struggling. One important aspect of this is monitoring for warning signs of depression and seeking early intervention when necessary.

Some common signs of depression in children include changes in mood, such as persistent sadness or irritability, a lack of interest in activities that they used to enjoy, changes in sleep patterns or appetite, and difficulty concentrating or making decisions.

If you notice any of these changes in your child, it is important to speak with a healthcare professional or mental health provider for further evaluation and treatment. Early intervention can be crucial in helping children to manage their symptoms and to get on the path to recovery.

Another important factor in preventing depression in children is providing support and resources for those who have experienced stress or trauma. This may include counseling, therapy, or other forms of support to help children cope with difficult experiences and build resilience. Children who have experienced significant stress or trauma may be at an increased risk for developing depression, so it is important to provide them with the necessary resources and support to help them navigate these challenges.

In addition to these measures, it is important to address any underlying medical or psychological conditions that may increase the risk for depression in children. This may include conditions such as anxiety, ADHD, or other mental health disorders, as well as physical health conditions that may affect a child's mood and well-being. By addressing these underlying conditions, it is possible to reduce the risk of depression and help children to lead healthy and fulfilling lives.

Finally, it is important to create a safe and supportive environment for children and to be aware of any changes in their behavior or mood that may indicate the need for further evaluation or treatment.

This may involve providing a stable and nurturing home environment, as well as being available to listen and offer support when needed. By taking these steps, we can help to prevent depression in children and ensure that they have the resources and support they need to thrive.

It is also worth noting that there are various treatment options available for children with depression, including medication, therapy, and lifestyle changes. Working with a healthcare professional or mental health provider can help to determine the most appropriate course of treatment for your child, based on their individual needs and circumstances. With the right support and resources, children with depression can learn to manage their symptoms and lead healthy, fulfilling lives.

The Importance of Addressing Childhood Depression

Childhood depression is a serious mental health condition that affects children and adolescents and can have a significant impact on their development, relationships, and overall well-being. It is characterized by persistent feelings of sadness, hopelessness, and a lack of interest in activities that were previously enjoyed.

Children with depression may also experience changes in appetite, sleep patterns, and energy levels, as well as difficulty concentrating, low self-esteem, and thoughts of self-harm or suicide. It is essential to recognize and address childhood depression as soon as possible in order to provide the necessary support and treatment for the child. Early intervention and treatment can not only alleviate the symptoms of the disorder but also prevent it from becoming more severe and improve the child's chances of making a full and complete recovery.

It is important for parents, caregivers, and other adults in the child's life to be aware of the signs and symptoms of childhood depression and to seek help if they are concerned about a child's mental health. Childhood depression can be caused by a variety of factors, including genetics, environmental stressors, and life events such as the loss of a loved one or bullying. Children who have experienced trauma, abuse, or neglect may also be at an increased risk for developing depression.

It is important for children with depression to receive treatment from a mental health professional, such as a psychologist or psychiatrist, who can develop a personalized treatment plan to address the child's specific needs. This may include therapy, medication, or a combination of both.

Treatment for childhood depression is most effective when it is comprehensive and tailored to the individual needs of the child. This may include a combination of therapy, medication, and other interventions such as educational support, social skills training, and family therapy. It is also important for the child to have a strong support system, including caring and supportive parents, teachers, and friends, who can provide emotional and practical support during the treatment process. With the right support and treatment, children with depression can learn to manage their symptoms and lead happy, healthy lives.

Recovering from depression is a journey that requires patience, persistence, and support. It is important to provide ongoing assistance for children with depression, as they may need additional help in managing their symptoms and developing healthy coping mechanisms.

This may involve continuing treatment with medication and psychotherapy, as well as creating a supportive and understanding environment at home and in school. Engaging in activities that promote mental health and well-being, such as exercise, socialization, and hobbies, can also be beneficial in supporting a child's recovery from depression.

Enlisting the support of a healthcare provider or mental health professional can be crucial in developing a comprehensive care plan that addresses the child's individual needs and helps to ensure their ongoing progress and well-being.

This may involve regular check-ins with the healthcare provider or mental health professional to assess the child's progress and make any necessary adjustments to the care plan. It may also involve seeking out additional resources, such as support groups or online resources, to provide additional support and guidance.

It is important to remember that recovery from depression is not a linear process, and there may be setbacks and challenges along the way. It is important to be patient and understanding, and to offer encouragement and support as the child works through these challenges. It may also be helpful to educate oneself on the signs and symptoms of depression, as well as strategies for managing and coping with the condition. With the right support and guidance, children with depression can learn to manage their symptoms and lead fulfilling, healthy lives.

www.ingramcontent.com/pod-product-compliance
Lightning Source LLC
Chambersburg PA
CBHW071549260726

48653CB00007BA/2598